OXFORD MEDICAL PUBLICATIONS

Continence Promotion in
General Practice

PRACTICAL GUIDES FOR GENERAL PRACTICE

Editorial Board

J. A. Muir Gray, Community Physician,
Oxfordshire Health Authority.
Ann McPherson, General Practitioner, Oxford.
Michael Bull, GP Tutor, Oxford.
John Tasker, GP Tutor, North Oxfordshire.

Continence Promotion in General Practice

Practical Guides for General Practice 13

by
NIGEL SMITH
Consultant Geriatrician
Department of Health Care of the Elderly
Queen's Medical Centre
Nottingham

MAGGIE CLAMP
General Practitioner
Radcliffe on Trent
Nottingham

Oxford   New York   Tokyo
OXFORD UNIVERSITY PRESS
1991

Oxford University Press, Walton Street, Oxford OX2 6DP

Oxford New York Toronto
Delhi Bombay Calcutta Madras Karachi
Petaling Jaya Singapore Hong Kong Tokyo
Nairobi Dar es Salaam Cape Town
Melbourne Auckland

and associated companies in
Berlin Ibadan

Oxford is a trade mark of Oxford University Press

Published in the United States
by Oxford University Press, New York

British Library Cataloguing in Publication Data
(Data available)

Library of Congress Cataloging in Publication Data
Smith, Nigel.
Continence promotion in general practice/by Nigel Smith, Maggie
Clamp.
    p.   cm.—(Practical guides for general practice: 13)
(Oxford medical publications)
Includes bibliographical references.
Includes index.
1, Urinary incontinence.   2. Fecal incontinence.   I. Clamp,
Maggie.   II. Title.   III. Series.   IV. Series: Oxford medical
publications.
[DNLM: 1. Health Promotion.   2. Patient Education.   3. Urinary
Incontinence—in old age.   4. Urinary Incontinence—therapy.   WI
PR141NK no. 13/ /WJ 146 S655c]
RC921.I5S63 1991   616.6'2—dc20   90-14369
ISBN 0–19–262043–6

Typeset by Cotswold Typesetting Limited, Cheltenham
Printed in Great Britain by
Dotesios Ltd, Trowbridge, Wilts

Preface

Urinary incontinence is a common, treatable symptom which causes great distress and inconvenience to the patient. We can no longer assume that it is due to ageing changes or irremediable damage at childbirth. In recent years, advances in urodynamics and therapeutics have opened up new opportunities for treatment of urinary incontinence at home, provided that the patient's symptoms are thoroughly evaluated.

This book explains how to identify the underlying pattern of bladder dysfunction and focuses on practical interventions which help the patient to recover continence. A *joint medical–nursing evaluation* is needed to characterize the patient's symptoms and probable diagnosis. Habit retraining, pelvic floor exercises, intermittent self-catheterization, and drug treatment can then be commenced. Clear advice is given about how to evaluate the effect of each intervention and when to seek further help. We have used the term 'continence promotion' to describe this process of evaluation and treatment. Throughout the book, the emphasis is on treatments which are available to the General Practitioner.

Nottingham   N. S.
August 1990   M. C.

Acknowledgements

We should like to thank Sister Hilary Oliver, Continence Adviser, Nottingham Health Authority and Professor Mark Castleden, Department of Geriatric Medicine, Leicester General Hospital for comments made in planning this book and Sue Broughton for assistance with typing.

Contents

1 What is urinary incontinence?

Incontinence is surprisingly difficult to measure. Although it is a symptom, few patients actually present and ask for treatment. Even patients with severe symptoms deny being incontinent, a term they associate with total lack of control or old age. They will agree, however, to having 'accidents', leakage or dampness. Asking 'Are you always dry?' or 'Do you have any trouble controlling your bladder?' sometimes provides more information than direct questioning about incontinence.

Doctors and nurses use a range of terms to describe incontinence without defining them clearly. The same patient may be described by different nurses as being 'Dry with toileting', 'Always wet', and 'Incontinent all the time'. Nurses are learning to assess their patients in more detail and particularly to keep a chart so that they can describe the patient as 'Visiting the toilet 10-15 times daily, having incontinence and urgency usually between 8 and 11 in the morning and always being dry overnight'. This type of information offers more scope for treatment and monitoring the response to therapy, and it depends on accurate recording of toileting and incontinence by means of a chart.

Urinary incontinence is involuntary leakage of urine resulting in a social or hygienic problem. Daily incontinence is as common as diabetes. Under 65, the prevalence is 1 in 20, and over 75 it rises to 1 in 12 among people living at home.

An average general practice of 2200 includes about 25 young people and 15 people over 75 living at home with significant urinary incontinence in addition to those in institutional care. These cases represent people with several episodes a week who are having to make adjustments to their life-style as a result, such as staying at home, toileting before going out, planning shopping trips or wearing pads. Most practices are likely to include a number of elderly people in rest homes, nursing homes, and hospitals, about half of whom are likely to have significant urinary incontinence.

Surveys reveal that between a half to three-quarters of incontinent patients are too embarrassed to consult the doctor or the nurse. Some patients are fatalistic and believe that nothing can be done to relieve their symptoms. Many of these patients have symptoms which severely disrupt their lives.

Most patients are otherwise fit. They include people with all patterns of urinary incontinence. They are influenced by the prevailing assumptions that incontinence is untreatable and unavoidable. Younger women often conceal their symptoms with sanitary towels, and even by staying at home and never taking holidays whilst trying to keep the truth from close relatives and friends.

Continence clinics have reported that about half of patients referred are completely cured and at least two-thirds improved.

The major factors in achieving success are a thorough history, detailed evaluation, and intensive follow-up.

The General Practitioner (GP) needs to be involved when a patient is treated for incontinence at home. Without the GP, no diagnosis is made and there is a danger of missing simple treatable conditions. There are many conditions which can be effectively identified and treated at home, so that hospital admission or clinic attendance can be avoided; those conditions are the subject of this book. The nurse is well placed to assess, chart, monitor, and advise the patient, but the treatment will not be complete without the GP being actively involved.

Simply providing pads and pants is not a way to use

nursing skills efficiently; every health centre or surgery could benefit from having one district nurse with particular skills in promoting continence. Many health authorities now run courses for district nurses and some are aiming to train all their community nurses in this way, so the need for GP involvement is urgent.

Most districts now have a continence adviser, who can advise district nurses and GPs on how to promote continence at home. A continence adviser is a nurse who has particular skills in continence promotion. He or she will have attended a course on continence promotion, and will have experience of joint medical-nursing evaluation of a range of conditions causing incontinence. The continence adviser has responsibilities in providing a *service to patients*, *teaching*, and *research*.

The **service** usually involves joint visits with the district nurse, a continence clinic, and intensive follow-up of a small case-load of patients. The emphasis is on advising the existing primary health-care team on continence promotion and incontinence management in the home, enabling the doctor and nurse to gain experience with a range of treatments which can be provided at home.

Continence advisers **teach** patients, relatives, carers, nurses, and other professional groups and have valuable resources for teaching techniques of continence promotion.

Research is important for continence advisers because we understand so little about how patients recover continence and because of the wealth of new materials and protective clothing for incontinence.

Continence advisers may be based in hospital or the community. Those based in hospital obviously have closer links with urological, gynaecological or geriatric services. Advisers accept direct referrals from GPs district nurses, hospital doctors, and patients themselves. They inform the GP of referrals of their patients, request background information, and send a summary of the findings. Patients are evaluated jointly by the doctor and nurse and in some instances undergo simple urodynamics (see below). The continence clinic may be run as part of the urology, gynaecology or geriatric service. Continence advisers are pleased to accept invitations to speak on promoting continence and managing incontinence.

Many health authorities employ specialist health visitors, who are experienced in toilet training, continence promotion, and incontinence management, for mentally and physically handicapped children.

Isolated urinary incontinence is rarely a symptom of serious disease. There is a great deal that can be done to identify the likely cause of incontinence so that the patient can be treated entirely at home.

Patients with urinary incontinence and other symptoms, such as urethral or bladder pain, haematuria, urinary retention, and uraemia, should be referred immediately for hospital investigation. When to refer patients with incontinence alone depends a lot on the patient's history and the practitioner's experience. Those patients who have failed to respond to 'common sense' management of their condition may benefit. Urodynamics will reveal the underlying bladder dysfunction, if any.

Urodynamics is measuring the pressure and volume of the bladder during filling and voiding. Saline or X-ray medium is run into the bladder and the resulting pressure changes can be observed. The test is normally carried out in an X-ray department by urologists or radiologists and takes about 30 minutes. Urodynamics is also called cystometry or videocystometry. Although the test is artificial and can create artefacts, it is the most accurate measure of the way the bladder works in daily life.

It is not always possible to make a diagnosis of bladder dysfunction after carrying out urodynamics. All series report some patients with evident symptoms whose urodynamic test reveals no abnormality. Urologists will sometimes advise empirical treatment for patients with typical symptoms, particularly pure stress incontinence.

The subject of this book is continence promotion, using methods that can be applied to the patient at home by the district nurse and GP working together. Continence promotion techniques include habit retraining, pelvic floor exercises, and intermittent self-catheterization.

Advanced continence promotion includes biofeedback, galvanic stimulation, hypnosis, and behavioural management. All these methods could be used at home, but the focus of this book is on common, basic techniques which can be applied to most patients in general practice.

2 What causes urinary incontinence?

At least 20 different conditions usually cause urinary incontinence. Some of these conditions, such as infections and glycosuria, can easily be identified and treated in general practice, while others will require specialist referral. As a first step, it is worth examining the abdomen, perineum, and urine for associated conditions:

Abdomen
   —constipation
   —pelvic mass: uterine myoma
                     ovarian mass
   —palpable bladder

Perineum
  —cystocele
  —tight foreskin
  —large inguinal hernia
  —uterine prolapse
  —*Candida* rash
  —prostatic hypertrophy
  —faecal impaction
  —atrophic vaginitis

Urine
  —glycosuria
  —urinary tract infection

It is always wise to take a midstream urine sample (MSU) from people with urinary incontinence, but although symptoms improve when an infection is treated, they often do not disappear altogether. Severe constipation can cause urinary incontinence; a loaded colon may exacerbate bladder instability or prevent normal bladder emptying. Faecal impaction is nearly always associated with urinary retention (see Chapters 3 and 9).

Urinary incontinence is also associated with a range of neurological disorders, most of which are easily identified:

- Stroke
- Dementia syndrome
- Parkinson's disease
- Multiple sclerosis
- Prolapsed lumbar disc
- Cervical spondylosis
- Spina bifida
- Spinal injury
- Diabetic autonomic neuropathy
- Poor mobility
- Reduced manual dexterity

Incontinence associated with these conditions is more

difficult to correct at home. Treatment of Parkinson's disease, for instance, rarely cures associated incontinence. For more details about neurological disorders and incontinence, see Chapter 8.

Characterizing the type of underlying bladder disorder, irrespective of its cause, helps to plan effective treatment. Three steps to characterize the type of bladder dysfunction which causes urinary incontinence:

1. Keep a frequency chart.
2. Do a standing stress test.
3. Measure post-voiding residual volume.

These three steps are also useful in those patients who have no evident cause for their incontinence. As a result, virtually all patients with urinary incontinence can be grouped as having three broad categories of bladder dysfunction (Table 1). This is extremely useful because each group has a different treatment which can be applied in general practice (see Chapter 4).

Table 2.1.   Patterns of bladder dysfunction causing incontinence

1. Unstable	2. Stress	3. Retention
Urgency and frequency	Dribbling on coughing	Continual leakage
	Positive stress test	Residual volume > 100 ml

The unstable bladder

People of all ages with all kinds of diseases can suffer from bladder instability. The bladder contracts unpredictably at relatively small volumes, resulting in urgency and having to rush to the toilet. Severity of symptoms often varies from day to day and particularly at different times of day, characteristically being worse in the early morning.

It is instinctive to try to contract the external sphincter and pelvic floor to prevent incontinence during unstable bladder contractions, but voluntary contraction cannot stop voiding once the micturition reflex is under way. The external urethral sphincter rapidly fatigues and cannot sustain urethral closure when the detrusor muscle contracts.

Patients who succeed in stopping mid-stream do so by inhibiting the detrusor contraction. This explains why some patients are unable to restart voiding when it has been interrupted. For identifying and treating bladder instability see Chapter 5.

Stress incontinence

Pelvic floor weakness occurs after childbirth in women and results in stress incontinence, that is leakage of urine on standing, coughing, sneezing, or any form of exertion.

In many cases, symptoms become more noticeable after the menopause as a result of ageing and hormonal changes. Stress incontinence alone frequently explains urinary incontinence in women in their eighties.

It is not easy to distinguish stress and urge incontinence. The two conditions commonly coexist, and both history and examination can be misleading. A 'standing stress test' aims to identify patients with symptomatic stress incontinence, the majority of whom will have 'genuine stress incontinence'. For an explanation of these terms, see Chapter 6.

Urinary retention

Urinary retention is much more frequent than used to be thought in both older men and women. Without checking a post-voiding residual volume, it is impossible to know if treatment failure could be due to a large, atonic bladder. Older women, particularly, are prone to developing a large, low-pressure bladder, which is difficult or impossible to identify on clinical examination.

Retention is vitally important because its management is different (anti-cholinergic agents are contra-indicated), and because of the dangers of recurrent infections and renal failure (if raised bladder pressure develops). For further details of retention and its treatment, see Chapter 7.

Post-micturition dribbling occurs after voiding in males of all ages. It seems to be due to pooling of urine between the internal and external urethral sphincter and failure of the normal 'milk-back' of urine into the bladder after voiding. It is often seen in patients with obstructive symptoms due to prostate hypertrophy, but it does not necessarily resolve with relief of the obstruction. Sitting down to pass urine may help and pressing upwards on the urethra, immediately posterior to the scrotum, after voiding. This can release the last few drops of urine which would otherwise leak out minutes later when the external urethral sphincter relaxes.

3   Approach to the patient

Encouraging patients to come forward with symptoms of incontinence takes time. Sometimes, the main battle is to overcome your own embarrassment. If you give your patients the chance to describe their bladder symptoms and their own response to them, you will probably find that more patients present and incontinence may emerge as an underlying symptom or fear in some long-standing surgery attenders. People with incontinence are often surprised to find they are not the only people in the world with the condition.

Spending time developing rapport will improve your results in getting people dry. You will hear patients say: 'No one has listened to me like this before' and 'I feel better already', after spending a few minutes taking a history. Imagine how you would feel after being incontinent in public: shame, loss of self-respect, depression—a feeling of total loss of control. Talking to someone about it can be very effective in beginning the process of recovery.

Every incontinent patient needs a *joint medical-nursing evaluation* before receiving any treatment; a detailed history, examination, and some simple tests to identify the pattern of bladder dysfunction.

A detailed history

Precipitating factors are important in incontinence: cough (stress), anxiety (urge), or continual incontinence (overflow). Does rain, a bus journey, the nearness of a toilet, or exertion make it worse? Does anything relieve the incontinence? Is it worse at a particular time of the day? Do patients use pads and are they effective? Many patients will have been using household materials, such as cut-up towels or sheets!

Has the patient had to make any change in shopping, inviting people round, holidays or going out since the symptoms began? Is sexual activity affected?

The history makes it possible to plan objectives. People often find their incontinence unmanageable at certain times of day. Someone with urgency and incontinence during the day and night may say they can cope with their symptoms provided that they do not have wet beds. In some cases this objective may be much easier to achieve than total dryness.

Examination

Abdominal
Several different conditions associated with urinary incontinence may be identified on abdominal examination:

- Constipation
- Pelvic mass
- Uterine myoma
- Ovarian mass
- Palpable bladder

Constipation can exacerbate the unstable bladder. Faecal impaction and pelvic masses are associated with retention of urine. Unfortunately, an enlarged bladder is not always palpable, especially when associated with obesity. Suprapubic pressure will sometimes elicit a feeling of urgency in patients with incomplete bladder emptying.

Perineal examination
Examination of the urethral meatus and vaginal and rectal examination may help in finding the cause of incontinence:

- Tight foreskin
- Large inguinal hernia
- Uterine prolapse
- Cystocele
- Atrophic vaginitis
- *Candida* rash
- Prostatic hypertrophy
- Faecal impaction

It is always embarrassing to miss a simple cause of urinary incontinence at the urethral meatus; a simple circumcision may be all that is needed. Large inguinal hernias are more problematic because they frequently present in multi-handicapped patients who would be a major anaesthetic risk. Uterine prolapse and cystocele are often found together, and are discussed in Chapter 6.

Some degree of perineal inflammation is common in patients with urinary incontinence. *Candida* infection is more likely in diabetics and is usually accompanied by itching and characteristic white patches. A high vaginal swab and culture will confirm the diagnosis.

Benign prostatic hypertrophy usually presents with hesitancy, frequency, and nocturia. Chapter 5 considers how obstructive symptoms can be differentiated from other bladder disorders.

Older people with faecal impaction almost invariably have urinary retention. Bladder emptying often recovers when the impaction is cleared. Patients that have a bed/chair existence at home or in residential care are very likely to develop periodic faecal impaction. Factors that help to prevent faecal impaction include:

- High fluid intake
- High-fibre diet
- High level of awareness of staff/relative

Urine

A mid-stream specimen of urine can easily be sent for culture and tested for glucose and blood in order to determine:

- Haematuria
- Glycosuria
- Urinary tract infection

Microscopic haematuria is seen in males with prostatic hypertrophy, in females during menstruation, and in both sexes during urinary tract infections. If there is no evident cause, refer the patient to a urologist for cystoscopy.

Glycosuria results in an osmotic diuresis which can precipitate incontinence in vulnerable patients. Improved control of blood glucose levels may rectify urinary complaints of diabetics.

Blood

In the elderly, incontinence may be a symptom of almost any disease. If you suspect a systemic cause, the patient should be referred to a geriatric outpatient clinic. Simple blood tests that could be carried out to exclude a metabolic or endocrine cause for incontinence are listed below:

- Urea and electrolytes
- Glucose
- Calcium
- Alkaline phosphatase

In many patients with urinary incontinence, the examination and investigations will be entirely normal. Carrying out a full examination reassures the patient that the local causes for incontinence have been investigated and that your have 'left no stone unturned'. You can then proceed to identify the pattern of the underlying bladder dysfunction.

4 Identifying the underlying bladder disorder

Three simple steps will reveal the pattern of the underlying bladder disorder in urinary incontinence: (1) keeping a frequency chart; (2) carrying out a standing stress test; (3) measuring post-voiding residual volume.

A frequency chart is easy to keep and in most cases the patients themselves or a relative can do it (Fig. 4.1). This is the first step towards improving the care of incontinent patients in general practice.

Keeping a chart has important benefits for patients. They frequently recognize that the incontinence has a pattern and that goals, such as extending dry periods, can be attained. It is natural for a patient who is dry overnight to wonder why he/she only has symptoms in the daytime.

Simply recording the time of voids and incontinence is worthwhile, but drinks, urine volumes, and any significant events in the day can also be recorded. Many health authorities publish their own fluid intake charts, and some manufacturers have printed charts specifically for recording continent status (see Appendix).

Patients' estimates of the severity of their symptoms are highly subjective; some patients with minor symptoms are very distressed and upset, whereas others seem to tolerate the most severe and inconvenient symptoms calmly and without complaint. This explains why a chart is so central for active treatment of urinary incontinence.

The chart which gives the most information is the frequency–volume chart (Fig. 4.2). The patient keeps a record of every visit to the toilet and the volume of urine passed (using a plastic jug), the number of episodes of

✓ = passed urine
C = cup of tea
W = wet

	Monday	Tuesday			
6am	✓				
7am	C	✓ C			
8am	✓	✓			
9am					
10am	W	C			
11am	✓✓ C	W			
12pm		✓ C			
1pm	W C	✓			
2pm					
3pm	✓				
4pm		✓ C			
5pm	✓				
6pm	✓ C	✓			
7pm		✓ C			
8pm					
9pm		✓			
10pm	✓ C	C			
11pm		✓			
12am					
1am		✓			
2am	✓				
3am					
4am					
5am					
Total	9	10			

Fig. 4.1. Frequency chart illustrating a patient with incontinence and low fluid intake.

	Monday	Tuesday			
6am	300				
7am		300			
8am	200 100	100			
9am	50 400	100 300			
10am		100			
11am	75(w) 250	150			
12pm	100	100			
1pm	100	150 250			
2pm	100	100 100			
3pm	400				
4pm	100	100(w) 250			
5pm	200	100			
6pm	100	150			
7pm		100			
8pm	75	150			
9pm		175 100			
10pm	100	100			
11pm	100				
12am		100			
1am	300				
2am					
3am					
4am					
5am					
Total	12× 1450	13× 1400			

Fig. 4.2. Frequency–volume chart illustrating a patient with frequency, reduced bladder capacity, incontinence, and fluid intake <1500 ml/day.

incontinence, the timing of drinks, and any other significant events in the day.

A patient who has a dry night and then passes 600 ml and is incontinent later in the day has a normal functional bladder capacity and the ability to inhibit bladder contractions through the night. This patient is very close to being dry all the time. Minor alterations in toileting times may be all that is needed.

On the other hand, a patient who never passes more than 100 ml has a very severely reduced bladder capacity. He or she should be referred to a urologist for cystoscopy because the chances of a bladder lesion, such as neoplasm, are increased. Recording urine volume also helps to identify those patients whose fluid intake is too low.

A frequency–volume chart also helps to identify objectives and the timing of medications.

There is nearly always a pattern to the incontinence. Usually it is worse in the morning: patients whose symptoms are maximal at 6 a.m. will be helped most by medications prescribed last thing at night. Some patients are only incontinent at night, and others only during the day. Findings such as these are often a surprise to the patient. The objective of treatment could be to reduce urgency when it occurs at inconvenient times, for instance, at work, or to control nocturnal frequency.

Finally, keeping a chart gives the patient an active part in his own assessment, encouraging him/her to think of possible causes, and underlining the idea that their symptoms may vary from week to week, and may even improve.

A week of charting is usually long enough to establish a baseline. In some cases, longer periods of observation may be needed. In nocturnal enuresis, for example, 3 or 4 weeks of charting may be needed to estimate the average number of wet beds per week, so that the effect of an intervention can be evaluated.

Standing stress test

Asking the patient to cough during examination of the perineum will generally reveal stress incontinence if it is present. Additionally, a *standing stress test* will identify a larger group of female patients with pelvic floor weakness. The patient stands, preferably with a full bladder, holds a tissue between her legs and coughs. If the tissue is moist, she has stress incontinence.

Asking the patient to contract her pelvic floor muscles during a pelvic examination 'as if she had diarrhoea and had to hold on' will show how strong the pelvic floor muscles are and how easily fatigued. It is also clear if the patient can accurately identify and contract the correct muscles.

Residual volume

This is the only way to exclude urinary retention in general practice. Patients of all ages and both sexes may have unrecognized retention of urine causing incontinence.

The patient is asked to empty the bladder and a disposable plastic catheter is inserted into the bladder, urine is drained off and the catheter is withdrawn. Patients with a residual volume of more than 100 ml have significant urinary retention.

Male and female length catheters for intermittent catheterization are available on NHS prescription, they are usually made of clear plastic and district nurses will often have used them during their work in the hospital.

The only reliable non-invasive method for estimating residual volume is *abdominal ultrasound*. Bladder volume is calculated from the area of the bladder on sagittal and transverse scans. A portable Bladderscan device offers GP-operated ultrasound in the surgery and at the patient's home (see appendix).

There are three common patterns of bladder dysfunction:

1. Unstable bladder (Chapter 5).
2. Stress incontinence (Chapter 6).
3. Urinary retention (Chapter 7).

Some patients will have more than one disorder—stress incontinence and bladder instability often occur together. A bladder which is unstable *and* retaining urine is particularly difficult to treat.

Once you have a clear picture of the pattern and severity of symptoms, you can explain your findings and management plan to the patient and offer a range of treatments, such as habit retraining, pelvic floor exercises, or modifying the drug regime.

Most patients can understand a simple explanation of the cause of their bladder disorder. Explaining the likely cause helps the patient to realize that he/she is not just incontinent but that they have a specific disorder of bladder filling or emptying which may respond to a variety of treatments. Sometimes, you may be able to offer the patient a choice of possible treatments for their symptoms. If the patient selects a treatment option, compliance will probably be greater and therefore success is more likely.

5 Treatment of bladder instability

Patients with *bladder instability* present with a combination of frequency, urgency, and incontinence and often agree when asked 'Do you have to rush to the toilet?' Many patients will say that sometimes they have incontinence with no warning at all. Common precipitants of unstable contractions include: standing, cold, rain, proximity to a toilet, thinking about it, and bumpy bus journeys. People often find that after shopping for two hours without voiding, returning home releases a powerful unstable contraction ('key-in-the-door incontinence').

Unstable contractions often result in heavy incontinence and can occur immediately after successful voiding. They are generally pain-free, but may be accompanied by a feeling of supra-pubic pain in catheterized patients and those with a combination of instability and retention ('detrusor sphincter dyssynergia', see below).

Symptoms of bladder instability are usually confined to certain times of the day only. Some patients only have frequency at work, others only have urgency and incontinence at night or during sexual intercourse.

Stable and unstable bladders

Anatomically there is no difference between an unstable and a normal bladder. The unstable bladder behaves differently because a loss of cortical inhibition allows the detrusor muscle to contract almost without warning. Continence is normally retained not by sphincters contracting, but by a lack of activity in the powerful detrusor muscle of the bladder wall. Someone with an unstable bladder would experience urgency or incontinence long before reaching a normal capacity of 400 ml.

The critical factor is the ability to postpone voiding once the need is perceived. Some otherwise asymptomatic individuals cannot help voiding involuntarily in the bath at home or in the swimming pool.

In many cases, life events seem to trigger a change from normal bladder function to instability. Psychological factors have a powerful influence over bladder function, as any examination candidate will report! People with urgency often describe themselves as having a 'weak bladder', implying a lifelong history of bladder instability. There may be some variation in the learning of bladder control, but this does not exclude the possibility of further learning or treatment.

Patients with bladder instability often have no detectable pathology either in the nervous system or the bladder. However, the unstable bladder does occur in patients with neurological conditions, such as multiple sclerosis or stroke. The unstable bladder is so common that it is likely to occur alongside many other conditions, such as constipation, diabetes, and arthritis in the elderly.

Patients commonly report that their symptoms are worse when they are anxious or upset. Some even experience incontinence if they get angry—a very frustrating symptom!

Fear of being incontinent can become a much larger problem to the patient than the actual incontinence itself. The result is withdrawal from social contact and elaborate attempts to conceal the symptoms. Patients become isolated and inward-looking so that paradoxically, when they consult a doctor, they find it a great relief to speak openly about their symptoms.

The unstable bladder is hardly ever an indication of serious disease, but it is embarrassing and disruptive. Patients are continually having to ask where the nearest toilet is, to remember to toilet themselves before going out, and know that an unexpected wait could be disastrous.

Treatment of the unstable bladder

All the conditions that we treat have a psychosomatic element to them; this explains why taking time to develop rapport, explain treatment, and follow progress achieves better results. In many cases the treatment is designed to help the patient to gain confidence and recover a feeling of self-control.

Explaining the nature of the condition is the first step in this process. Two alternative treatments for bladder instability can be easily applied in general practice:

1. Habit retraining.
2. Anti-cholinergic drugs.

However, many otherwise fit people are understandably unwilling to take tablets for their incontinence.

Habit retraining is not as regimented as bladder drill or two-hourly toileting, it is more flexible. Habit retraining is an individualized plan of toileting and drinking adjusted according to response.

Plan of habit retraining
1. Baseline assessment.
2. Define objectives.
3. Plan an intervention.
4. Evaluate its effect.

Retraining requires intensive follow-up which is best carried out by the district nurse. It relies on the nurse's skill, experience, and confidence. Most continence advisers are pleased to assist in the management of individual cases and to introduce district nurses to this technique. Training courses are run in most districts and deal specifically with continence promotion in the community.

Baseline assessment involves identifying the times of day when incontinence is particularly likely to occur. The pattern and severity of frequency, urgency, and incontinence will be evident after a week of charting.

Define objectives means deciding with the patient which symptoms are most important or annoying to them, and setting a realistic objective for the following week.

Plan an intervention This may involve an increase in drinking, more frequent toileting at particular times of day, or a change in the patient's daily routine.

Once they have achieved dryness by more frequent toileting, patients are asked to extend the time between toileting. Afficianados of this approach work in intervals of a quarter of an hour. At first, it is probably more realistic to increase the intervals by 30-minute steps and to choose patients to work with who have a functional bladder capacity of at least 400 ml.

Evaluate its effect This step is often left out, but it is at the heart of all therapy. What has the intervention achieved? If the honest answer is 'Nothing', then an alternative intervention can be made without losing the patient's confidence.

Success depends on developing rapport with the patient. Recovery relies on the ability to re-learn the unconscious process of inhibiting a detrusor contraction Success rates of over 60 per cent have been reported among patients with straightforward bladder instability.

Most patients have reduced their fluid intake in an attempt to diminish their symptoms, but many find that the effect is exactly the opposite. Sometimes increasing fluid intake is all that is needed for the patient to recover continence.

Occasionally, charting will reveal a heavy tea or coffee drinker. Theophylline derivatives are diuretics and excessive tea or coffee intake is a rare cause of urinary incontinence.

The skills of habit retraining can be rapidly learned through joint visits by a district nurse and a continence adviser. Although it does require time and effort, the rewards are immediate and there are potential savings in having less pads to deliver!

The management of the unstable bladder in stroke or

multiple sclerosis is often identical. However, the neuro-logical deficit can create difficulties with co-ordination, communication or mobility.

Drugs and urinary incontinence

Some drugs that can exacerbate bladder instability are:

- Loop diuretics
- Benzodiazepines, e.g. nitrazepam

There have been many advances in drugs for urinary incontinence and many of the older drugs are no longer used, e.g. emepromium, flavoxate, and propantheline are used much less nowadays. Imipramine, terodiline, and oxy-butynin are often used to control symptoms of urgency and frequency. The powerful detrusor muscle is stimulated by parasympathetic fibres releasing the neuro-transmitter acetylcholine; all three drugs have anti-cholinergic effects:

Drugs to relieve bladder instability
- Imipramine
- Terodiline
- Oxybutynin

Imipramine, a tricyclic anti-depressant, has had the longest use. Its long half-life in the elderly enables small doses of 10–25 mg to be used on a once-a-day basis. At this dosage, troublesome side-effects, such as drowsiness and postural hypotension, are less likely to occur. The therapeutic effect is generally evident in the first week.

The main drawback of using imipramine is the occur-rence of unwanted anti-cholinergic side-effects, such as a dry mouth, blurred vision, tachycardia, and facial flushing. Nearly all patients notice a dry mouth, so it is worth warning them in advance of this particular side-effect.

Terodiline is a combined anti-cholinergic agent and calcium channel blocker. Its calcium antagonist action is selective to the bladder so that heart rate and blood pressure are not normally affected at recommended doses of 12.5–25 mg, twice daily. Its half-life is around 60 hours and a steady state is reached after 10–14 days of administration. The half-life is considerably prolonged in ill elderly patients for whom the lower dose is recommended. Side-effects, such as dry mouth, tremor, and headaches appear to be dose-related: occasionally, gastro-intestinal upset, tachycardia or pruritis may be seen.

Oxybutynin is an anti-cholinergic agent and smooth muscle relaxant, and has similar side-effects to imipramine. It is unlicensed and not listed in the British National Formulary and can only be prescribed in the United Kingdom on a named-patient basis. It is generally prescribed at a dosage of 5–10 mg three times a day, but if symptoms are limited to the morning, 5 mg once a day may be all that is required.

Imipramine, *terodiline*, and *oxybutynin* have been shown to shift the balance towards bladder stability in patients with unstable contractions. Studies have shown a trend towards higher bladder capacities and less frequent unstable contractions on testing; all three are more effective than placebo in enabling the patient to recover continence. If the treatment is effective, most patients will tolerate the anti-cholinergic side-effects. Postural hypotension, facial flushing, skin rashes, and drowsiness seen with higher doses of imipramine are less well tolerated. Now that acetylcholine is known to be depleted in Alzheimer's disease, added caution is needed when prescribing anti-cholinergics for older people with mild forgetfulness or early dementia syndrome.

Imipramine is maximally effective 6 to 8 hours after the dose is taken, so patients with nocturnal or early morning symptoms can take it at 8 or 10 p.m. and may avoid the most troublesome side-effects, such as a dry mouth, by sleeping through them. If a patient fails to respond to one agent, it may still be worth prescribing an alternative agent because their modes of action and side-effect profiles differ.

It may be worth withdrawing the treatment after two to three months because sometimes medical treament interrupts a vicious circle and the patient can gain enough confidence to manage entirely without the tablets. If symptoms recur, the treatment can easily be restarted.

Diuretics and incontinence

In older people, chronic ankle oedema has many causes other than congestive heart failure: sleeping in a chair, reduced mobility, osteoarthritis of knees and hips or previous deep venous thrombosis can cause this condition.

Dehydration, secondary to diuretics, can be dangerous with the risk of falls, drowsiness, and peripheral infarcts. Nowadays, it is possible to introduce angiotensin-converting-enzyme inhibitors for patients with heart failure who become incontinent when prescribed loop diuretics.

Very occasionally, diuretics can be helpful in treating incontinence. Some elderly people lose the normal pattern of daytime voiding and a frequency–volume chart will reveal that they pass a larger volume of urine at night, resulting in nocturnal frequency and enuresis. A short-acting loop diuretic prescribed in the morning reverses this pattern and can contribute to the recovery of night-time continence. When this happens in the course of a stroke, the diuretics can often be withdrawn as the patient recovers.

Benzodiazepines and incontinence

Older people are particularly sensitive to the sedative side-effects of nitrazepam, which may cause nocturnal and morning incontinence. Alternatives include chlormethiazcle, lormetazepam, and triazolam.

Drawbacks to drug therapy
1. Anti-cholinergic side-effects.
2. Precipitating retention.
3. Non-compliance.

Retention of urine is a potentially serious complication of using agents with anti-cholinergic side-effects. For this reason, it is important to exclude urinary retention in patients whose symptoms have been unchanged or become worse on drug treatment. High-pressure retention, which occurs in prostatic hypertrophy and spina bifida, can damage the kidneys. Low-pressure retention causes recurrent urinary tract infections.

Obstruction is common in males but almost unknown in females. A weak, acontractile bladder occurs with increasing frequency among elderly people and is the main cause of retention in females. Patients with diabetes and multiple sclerosis are likely to have a poorly co-ordinated voiding reflex and present with a combination of instability and retention which can be extremely difficult to manage in general practice.

Detrusor sphincter dyssynergia

This is a form of bladder instability in which the co-ordination between the detrusor and the urethral sphincter is lost. Normally, a bladder contraction is characterized by electrical silence in the internal urethral sphincter. In dyssynergia, a segment of the urethra contracts during voiding to cause incomplete emptying.

Symptoms, such as a feeling of incomplete emptying, dribbling incontinence, voiding twice in quick succession ('double voiding'), suggest a voiding disorder. The only way to be sure is to measure the residual volume before and after commencing treatment.

Nocturnal enuresis

The most common cause of persistent bed-wetting is bladder instability. Although it is generally associated with children, enuresis usually emerges as a problem in 20–30-year-olds who have to stay away from home or start a new relationship. There is no correlation with deep sleep: incontinence occurs during rapid-eye-movement sleep. Primary nocturnal enuresis is commonly associated with a traumatic childhood, but may still respond to simple measures. The following are treatments for nocturnal enuresis in adults:

1. Anti-cholinergic drugs.
2. Pad alarms.
3. Hypnosis.
4. DDAVP.

Initial treatment for children is a star chart and a tangible reward for a series of dry nights. For adults, a *pad alarm* system can be surprisingly effective. The patient will need to wear a night-dress or pyjamas as well as a pad and pants. The battery-powered alarm clips on to the night clothes or fits into a pocket. Auditory, tactile, or visual alarms are available. A sensor which responds to the presence of small amounts of water is fitted inside the pad (Fig. 5.1).

When the patient voids, the sensor activates the alarm, which rings, vibrates, or flashes to alert the patient. Success depends on a working alarm which wakes the patient and

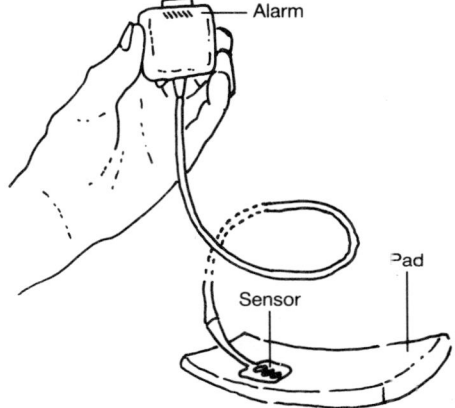

Fig. 5.1.   A pad alarm system. The alarm clips on to the pyjamas or night-dress and the sensor fits into an incontinence pad.

is used consistently. The brain is able to re-learn the ability to postpone voiding during sleep, or become more sensitive when voiding is imminent.

Bed-wetting is a habit which can be corrected using hypnosis. Techniques include ego-strengthening and direct symptom removal. Rapport and a willing, co-operative subject are central to a successful outcome.

DDAVP is a synthetic form of Anti-Diuretic Hormone (ADH) which can be given intra-nasally as drops or as a spray, 20 μg at night. It concentrates the urine and so reduces nocturnal urine production. It has a prolonged action and none of the vasoconstrictor actions of natural ADH. However, it should be used cautiously in the presence of heart disease, asthma, epilepsy or migraine. It may have a place in the treatment of adults with enuresis if all other treatments have failed or if a dry night is crucially important. Its main drawbacks are its expense and the present route of administration.

6 Treatment of stress incontinence

Patients with stress incontinence are likely to have dribbling incontinence, especially on lifting, coughing or exerting. On examination, a standing stress test is positive. Leakage on standing or coughing can be due to unstable detrusor contractions, so urologists reserve the term 'genuine stress incontinence' for patients whose urodynamic study reveals leakage of urine without a rise in detrusor pressure.

There may be no evidence of associated uterine prolapse. Prolapse and stress incontinence occur independently and treatment of prolapse often has no effect on the incontinence. The Stamey procedure is an example of a surgical technique specifically designed to raise the bladder neck and so correct stress incontinence; anterior vaginal repair does not appear to improve symptoms.

A lax anterior vaginal wall can sometimes cause urgency because the normal urethral closure mechanism is distorted. This may explain why some women with cystocele have a combination of stress and urge incontinence.

Atrophic vaginitis is associated with both stress incontinence and an 'irritable bladder'. This is because, in the absence of oestrogens, urethral closure pressure is lower and the trigone area of the bladder becomes inflamed, just like the vaginal wall.

Topical oestrogen creams, such as dienoestrol, are highly effective in reversing the changes due to oestrogen deficiency. Local application of water-permeable creams enables a small dose to be used and so reduces the side-effects. Patients who are unwilling to apply a cream can take ethinyloestradiol 10 μg daily. Treatment is usually continued for three months and can be repeated as needed.

About 5 per cent of women of all ages have significant stress incontinence. Prolonged labour and multiparity are major risk factors, but stress incontinence also occurs in women who have not had children.

Ring pessaries may relieve symptoms due to uterine prolapse, but they rarely help stress incontinence. Furthermore, many elderly women cannot tolerate them.

Stress and urge incontinence may occur during sexual activity and so affect personal relationships. Try to give your patients time to describe these effects and their own reactions of fear or embarrassment.

Treatment

- Pelvic floor exercises
- Cones
- Interferential therapy
- Surgery, e.g. Stamey procedure

Pelvic floor exercises Pelvic examination will reveal the strength and stamina of the pelvic floor muscles and will also establish if the patient can identify them correctly. Exercises can be arranged either through local physiotherapy services or via the continence adviser. Total cure is unlikely, but symptoms often improve enough for patients to return to a more active life, and avoid the need for surgery. Improvement can be expected even in 90- or 100-year-olds.

The underlying reason for stress incontinence appears to be damage to nerves and muscles during vaginal delivery, sometimes aggravated by ageing changes. There are excellent leaflets available which explain to patients how the exercises work and how often to do them (see Appendix). Patients are often surprised to hear that childbirth can result in symptoms much later in life.

It is possible to demonstrate a training effect in people of all ages. Speed of response and power of contraction can both be increased by exercise. The explanation lies in physiological changes in muscle fibres and their nerve and blood supplies. A small change in power may have a great effect on symptoms.

Most patients are able to learn to contract the levator ani and pubococcygeus muscles without contracting the gluteal muscles. They can then practice the exercises at, for example, the bus stop without being noticed! Keeping a chart of incontinent episodes will reveal the response to treatment.

Weighted cones are gaining in popularity. A series of graduated cones of steadily increasing weights is used; the patient is instructed to place a cone in the vagina, to stand up and retain the cone for a certain interval.

Results using this technique seem to be better than with pelvic floor exercises. It is clear when the patient is exercising the correct muscles and their progress is easily followed. The cones are available at chemists' shops and via some physiotherapy departments.

Interferential therapy Physiotherapists can provide interferential treatment which concentrates an electrical field around the pelvic floor. This causes the muscles to contract in people who are unable to contract their pelvic floor muscles voluntarily. This treatment is used sometimes for patients with multiple sclerosis and stress incontinence.

If a woman fails to respond to pelvic floor exercises, retention of urine needs to be excluded before referring to a gynaecologist for corrective surgery.

Stress incontinence rarely occurs in men.

Causes of stress incontinence in males
- Overflow incontinence in urinary retention
- Post-operative damage to the urethral sphincter

The internal urethral sphincter can be damaged following surgery, particularly when the prostate gland is malignant. The result is either stress incontinence, or in severe cases, continuous incontinence. Many patients can make the most of their remaining muscle function with pelvic floor exercises.

7 Management of urinary retention

Incontinence may be the only sign of retention. Patients characteristically have dribbling incontinence or stress incontinence. Frequency and double voiding can occur, i.e. voiding twice in quick succession. Some patients report a feeling of incomplete emptying of the bladder and sometimes supra-pubic pressure will elicit a feeling of bladder fullness, but an enlarged bladder is often not palpable.

Many of these signs and symptoms are unreliable and a post-voiding residual volume remains the most sensitive method in detecting urinary retention. Retention predisposes to recurrent urinary tract infection over-distends the bladder wall, and may be associated with raised bladder pressure.

If retention is causing symptoms, then the main aim of treatment becomes complete emptying of the bladder at voiding. Normal bladder function is much more likely to return if the bladder empties fully. Asymptomatic retention is, however, quite common in the elderly, especially amongst women, and requires no specific treatment.

Patterns of urinary retention
- Obstruction
- Acontractility
- Detrusor sphincter dyssenergia

Obstruction

The commonest cause of retention in males is prostatic hypertrophy. Men often develop an obstructive uropathy, with the danger of progressive renal failure due to bilateral hydronephrosis. The obstructed bladder tends to develop unstable features, making the differential diagnosis even more difficult. Obstruction is rare in females.

Acontractility

This is more common in older people. A weak, inefficient detrusor fails to empty the bladder. The urinary flow rate is reduced and the detrusor fails to contract during filling and voiding.

Prostatic size on rectal examination is a poor predictor of obstruction. A urine flowmeter which identifies patients with lower than normal flow rates is a more sensitive guide. Using a Valsalva manoeuvre or pressing the lower abdomen to empty the bladder, are both suggestive of a voiding disorder.

If retention persists once constipation has been relieved, a variety of treatments can be used:

- Stop drugs with anti-cholinergic side-effects
- Administer drugs which facilitate bladder emptying
- Intermittent catheterization
- Permanent catheter

Many drugs with anti-cholinergic side-effects are capable of exacerbating urinary retention, e.g.:

- Tricyclic anti-depressants
- Phenothiazines
- Phenytoin
- Propantheline
- Hydralazine
- Anti-arrhythmics, such as disopyramide

Drugs which facilitate bladder emptying

These include cholinergic agents to increase the power of the detrusor and alpha-1 adrenergic blockers to relax the urethral sphincter. The main drawbacks to treatment are side-effects and failure to relieve retention.

Cholinergic agents can cause blurred vision, dizziness, while the adrenergic blockers cause postural hypotension and tachycardia. Currently, selective alpha-1 adrenergic blockers are the most promising area of study. Drugs such as indoramin improve the flow rate and symptoms of male patients awaiting surgery for prostatic obstruction. Females have few alpha receptors at the bladder neck and a poorly developed internal urethral sphincter, so adrenergic agents are unlikely to work.

Intermittent and permanent catheterization

Intermittent catheterization is one of the most exciting developments in continence promotion. Many of the drawbacks of permanent catheters can be avoided simply by draining the bladder two or more times daily. Increasingly, urologists and geriatricians are making use of intermittent catheterization as an alternative to a permanent device (Table 7.1). Management of a permanent catheter is discussed in Chapter 11.

Table 7.1. Comparison of intermittent catheterization and permanent catheter in the management of urinary retention

Permanent catheter	Intermittent catheterization
Frequently block, bypass or fall out	Keeps the patient dry
All catheters infected at 1 month	Urinary tract infection easily treated
Foreign body; residual volume sustains infections	
Catheter blocking, bypass and displacement need medical/nursing time	Once trained, the patient can manage their own self-catheterization
Unsuitable for severely cognitively impaired patients; urethral trauma	Demands good hand–eye co-ordination, motivation, and cognitive function

It involves the patient, a relative or a nurse inserting a disposable plastic catheter to empty the bladder once, twice or many times a day. Some patients never pass urine in the normal way, so the bladder can be emptied once or twice a day. Other patients pass urine normally but would be incontinent if their bladders were allowed to accumulate a large volume of urine.

It is surprising how many male and female patients find they are able to use the technique. When the alternative is a permanent catheter, many patients would rather continue their sex life and avoid wearing a bag that continually slides down, quite apart from the constant discomfort of a tube in the bladder and urethra.

All patients with long-term catheters develop significant bacteriuria which sometimes results in life-threatening gram-negative septicaemia. Indwelling catheters are also associated with local abscesses, calculi, and urethral stricture. Social life is dramatically affected because of the embarrassment and inconvenience of the catheter and a normal sex life is virtually impossible.

Using an intermittent catheter does not entirely avoid abscesses, stricture or infections, but complications appear to be relatively rare. An intermittent catheter can be a way of training the bladder; the voiding reflex may recover when the bladder is emptied regularly and the harmful effects of over-distension are removed.

In young disabled people, it may be a way of managing incontinence without resorting to major surgery, such as cystoplasty (creating a new bladder), ileal drainage or an artificial sphincter.

All the patient needs is the manual dexterity to put a catheter into the urethra and the mental ability to understand the technique, a bladder capacity of over 100 ml, and a urethra free of stricture.

Any experienced nurse can demonstrate the technique of clean intermittent self-catheterization. The area around the meatus is cleaned to prevent pubic hairs from being advanced with the catheter into the bladder. Female patients often begin by using a mirror to find the urethral meatus, but many patients find it easier to use palpation. A plastic catheter is inserted into the bladder and the urine is collected and measured if necessary. Several different makes of disposable Nelaton catheters are available on NHS prescription. Most patients use the same catheter for a week at a time and clean it by washing it through with tap water and drying it out thoroughly.

Patients are warned about the early signs of bladder infections, such as bladder pain, frequency, and pyrexia. Some urologists provide their patients with antibiotics to take in the event of developing symptoms. Others advise taking an antibiotic, such as trimethoprim 200 mg daily during intermittent catheterization, but this is by no means universally agreed.

Children with spina bifida have been catheterizing

themselves for many years quite safely by using a 'clean' procedure. Sterile precautions are expensive and unnecessary. Organisms in the distal urethra are advanced into the bladder, but in retention, the major risk factor is the substrate presented by the large residual volume. Removing the substrate shifts the balance against infection. Although infections occur in patients using intermittent self-catheterization they seem to be less frequent than among patients in chronic retention.

Treatments can be prescribed for patients on intermittent self-catheterization which would otherwise be impossible because of the risks of aggravating retention. Anti-cholinergics may reduce urge incontinence in patients who have a combination of urgency and incomplete bladder emptying. Multiple sclerosis is a common example of a condition in which retention and urgency often coexist. Patients with a paraplegic form of the disease can catheterize themselves and a husband can sometimes learn to catheterize his wife.

8 Neurological causes of incontinence

Stroke

Drowsiness, aphasia, and poor mobility are all signs of a major stroke, and are commonly associated with incontinence. Causes of incontinence after stroke include:

- Impaired conscious level
- Sensory deficit, including hemianopia

- Perceptual deficit
- Aphasia
- Poor mobility
- Unrecognized epilepsy

The mechanism may be through disrupting the normal inhibitory pathways to the sacral micturition centre or by disturbing continent behaviour (see Table 8.1). This complex sequence of steps can be affected at several points after a stroke.

Table 8.1. Continent behaviour

In order to stay dry, a dependent patient needs to:
  −appreciate the need to void
  −communicate need to carer
  −be motivated
  −be able to weight bear
  −assist in transferring on to commode/toilet
  −be able to undress
  −delay voiding until the appropriate time
  −initiate voiding voluntarily

Loss of a normal body image, denial of any deficit, and inattention to one side (varieties of perceptual deficit) can be more disabling than evident motor loss.

The natural history of stroke is recovery. However severe their disability is, a sizeable proportion of stroke patients will recover continence. It is important to exclude common co-incidental causes, such as constipation, infection, prostatic hypertrophy or pelvic floor weakness.

Urodynamic studies reveal that the most common underlying bladder abnormality after stroke is the unstable bladder. Therefore, having excluded other causes, including retention, patients can be treated for bladder instability with habit retraining or anti-cholinergic agents.

Although incontinence is a poor prognostic sign, it is

more practical to look for 'good signs', so that you are alert for the early signs of recovery in your patients. Good prognostic signs after stroke are as follows:

- Recent stroke
- First stroke
- Insight into the deficit
- Alert, responsive patient
- Ability to copy a simple design
- Younger age group
- Early recovery of power and sitting balance

Recovery of continence commonly occurs spontaneously in stroke and for this reason it is important to continually review the need for an indwelling catheter. Evidence is accumulating that continence is a crucial factor affecting patient morale after stroke and that recovery of continence is associated with more rapid rehabilitation.

Dementia syndrome

Dementia is global impairment of cognitive function: speech; thought; memory; insight; self-care; and intelligence. The term 'dementia syndrome' includes many different diagnoses. The conditions where both dementia and urinary incontinence occur include:

- Alzheimer's disease
- Multi-infarct dementia
- Alcohol-induced brain damage
- Post-traumatic: head injury, encephalitis
- Normal pressure hydrocephalus

Urinary incontinence is seen in all forms of dementia and may be part of the syndrome of loss of motivation, disinhibition, and lack of insight. Important causes to recognize are depression and co-incidental disease.

Patients with normal pressure hydrocephalus dementia

have early gait disturbance and incontinence. They often neglect their self-care and walk with an 'apraxic' gait: feet 'glued' to the floor, taking lots of tiny steps with feet wide apart or reaching forwards for support just out of reach. Patients with these symptoms should be referred to the psycho-geriatrician or neurologist for assessment and possibly a computerized tomography (CT) scan.

Normal pressure hydrocephalus is the most common cause of reversible dementia. It is due to abnormal cerebrospinal fluid (CSF) dynamics and can follow subarachnoid haemorrhage, craniotomy or may be idiopathic. Studies of CSF pressure may confirm the diagnosis. Treatment is to insert a shunt to relieve the pressure—recovery can be dramatic. Obstructive hydrocephalus can also present subacutely in the elderly with self-neglect, incontinence, and gait disorder.

Faced with a patient with dementia syndrome and incontinence, the first essentials are to exclude organic disease, constipation associated with low fluid intake, and reduced physical activity. Regular bulk laxatives may help.

Relatives and carers will need to be immensely patient in explaining the way to the toilet and avoiding any disturbance to the normal routine. Rewards, such as human contact, may help to reinforce continent behaviour.

The most practical support is in anticipating a breakdown in the carers before it takes place by planning the use of day-centres, relief care in rest homes, night-sitters or psycho-geriatric referral.

Poor mobility and dementia syndrome are often associated with incontinence, but some patients are incontinent at home but consistently dry in hospital. Access to the toilet may be easier, nurses may be able to offer regular toileting to prevent incontinence, or at home there may be a dependent relationship, in which a carer provides more help than is strictly needed so that the patient falls into the dependent 'invalid' role.

Older women are often understandably reluctant to use a commode in the front room, and the thought of asking a relative or carer to empty a chemical toilet is often repulsive. If the patient is not requesting help for his or her incontinence, treatment must focus on how to limit the consequences and control other factors such as constipation.

The term 'Diogenes syndrome' has been applied by psycho-geriatricians to elderly people living at home in a state of extreme self-neglect, often incontinent and immune to the consequences, eating very little and refusing to accept help of any sort. Characteristically, they are cognitively otherwise completely normal. People with these features can be extremely difficult to help. On the other hand, urinary incontinence is a relatively late occurrence in senile dementia of Alzheimer type. When it occurs in the first year of dementia syndrome, the diagnosis of Alzheimer's disease should be questioned.

Finding an effective system to contain the symptoms, such as pads and pants, can also help if the patient is able to co-operate.

Other neurological disorders

Many neurological conditions can be associated with urinary incontinence:

- Parkinson's disease
- Multiple sclerosis (MS)
- Prolapsed lumbar disc
- Cervical spondylosis
- Spina bifida
- Spinal injury
- Diabetic autonomic neuropathy
- Poor mobility
- Reduced manual dexterity

In multiple sclerosis (MS), disturbance of cortical and

spinal pathways causes incontinence, although low fluid intake and constipation can still be important.

The underlying bladder disorder may be the unstable bladder, retention or a combination of the two: the three patterns occur in approximately equal proportions.

As MS is often a progressive condition, there is a constant need to evaluate the effect of therapy. The most difficult group of MS patients to treat are those with retention and bladder instability. Their combination of frequency and voiding disorder can be resistant to treatment either with frequent self-catheterization or anti-cholinergic agents.

Typically, male patients with loss of co-ordination between the detrusor and urethra also suffer sexual difficulties such as retrograde ejaculation.

Incontinence in diabetes may be due to glycosuria or diabetic autonomic neuropathy. In this condition, urgency and retention commonly coexist so that anti-cholinergics alone are often ineffective.

Spinal injuries and spina bifida commonly result in urinary retention and urologists are keen to avoid permanent catheters because of progressive renal damage due to recurrent infections. Some patients in both groups can be treated effectively with a penile sheath Patients with a high-pressure retention need either a surgical procedure to reduce bladder pressure or a catheter.

It is possible to implant an inflatable cuff around the urethra, filled by a reservoir under the skin (artificial urinary sphincter). The procedure is used, but it is very expensive and needs to be combined with a procedure to reduce outflow resistance.

9 Faecal incontinence

Faecal incontinence is often the factor which decides whether an elderly disabled patient can be managed at home by his/her own family or has to be admitted to a nursing home.

'Faecal incontinence' means involuntary leakage of faeces causing a social or hygienic problem. Like urinary incontinence, it may have local, rectal or neurological causes, or result from the patient's general condition. At an early stage, examination may reveal a treatable cause.

Is it faecal incontinence?

Faecal staining can sometimes be confused with incontinence if the patient has extreme anxiety about being incontinent. This is particularly likely to develop in a carer who has looked after a husband or mother with faecal incontinence. The use of a chart provides a measure of the frequency and severity of the incontinence as a baseline. Additional information about frequency of defaecation and consistency of stool can help to identify diarrhoea.

Inappropriate defaecation and faecal smearing are essentially behavioural disorders seen in association with self-neglect in dementia syndrome and very occasionally when a husband or wife is unnecessarily dependent.

The most important condition to identify is constipation.

Risk factors for constipation
- Low fluid intake

- Low-fibre diet
- Reduced mobility
- Anorexia
- Constipating drugs: anti-depressants; iron

Paradoxically, diarrhoea is commonly associated with severe constipation. This is because hard stool becomes impacted in the rectum and bacterial action and mucus production result in a loose, watery, offensive stool: 'overflow incontinence'.

Abdominal examination will often reveal a mass, usually in the left iliac fossa caused by a sigmoid colon dilated with faeces. Occasionally, the mass is in the right iliac fossa and difficult to distinguish from caecal carcinoma. Treatment with enemas and laxatives resolves both the mass and the change in bowel habit.

Rectal examination identifies faecal impaction, which usually demands treatment with enemas in immobile elderly patients. Faecal impaction can present as an acute abdomen or with vomiting and anorexia: rectal examination provides the diagnosis.

Faecal incontinence associated with diarrhoea may be a symptom of gastro-intestinal disease (Table 9.1). Investigation by proctoscopy, sigmoidoscopy, biopsy, stool culture, and barium enema is indicated. If no cause is found, some patients respond to an empirical course of rectal steroid enemas, such as Colifoam.

Table 9.1.   Causes of diarrhoea and faecal incontinence

Ulcerative colitis	Autonomic neuropathy
Non-specific proctitis	(e.g. Parkinson's disease,
Steatorrhoea	diabetes)
(e.g. bacterial overgrowth)	Colonic villous adenoma
Salmonella infection	Irritable bowel syndrome
Pseudo-membranous colitis	Amyloidosis

Faecal incontinence of formed stool may result from ano-rectal conditions:

- Denervated rectum
- Unstable rectum
- Haemorrhoids
- Anal stricture

Denervation may be associated with an 'adult megacolon' syndrome with the entire colon outlined by bowel gas on plain abdominal X-ray, and recurrent bouts of abdominal distension and sigmoid volvulus. If a flatus tube is passed early at home, admission and even operation may be avoided.

The unstable rectum is analogous to the unstable bladder: the rectum contracts unpredictably so that the patient has no warning of defaecation. The explanation lies in loss of the normal inhibition of rectal emptying.

Preventing severe constipation can be extremely difficult and involves using a pragmatic combination of agents which prove to be effective for that particular patient.

Bowel regime

A bowel regime consists of any combination of agents (Table 9.2) and is designed to establish a manageable

Table 9.2.   Components of a bowel regime

Constipating agents	Bulk laxatives
−codeine phosphate	−bran
Osmotic laxatives	−methyl cellulose
−lactulose	−ispaghula husk
−dioctyl succinate	Suppositories
−magnesium sulphate	−glycerol
Stimulant laxatives	−bisacodyl
−senna	Enemas
−bisacodyl	−Micralax
−sodium picosulphate	−phosphate

pattern of bowel emptying in patients with intractable faecal incontinence. In some cases, carers and relatives are prepared to look after the patient at home provided the bowel regime is successful.

10 Containing symptoms

Nowadays there is much more variety in the design of pads and pants. More resources go into the testing of new materials and better designs. There is a great need to match the patient's needs to the appropriate design. Manufacturers are continually adapting and developing the design of pads and pants, so even recent comparative studies may not relate to current designs available.

Some of the most detailed comparisons of pads and pants are listed in the Bibliography. A complete directory of aids and appliances for incontinence is published by the Association of Continence Advisors.

Finding a suitable system to contain incontinence demands an individual approach, taking into account each patient's needs and preferences. It is often helpful to demonstrate a range of designs so that each patient can choose one to suit their own particular needs.

Personal advice from a nurse who recognizes the advantages and disadvantages of each system is vital to the efficient use of pads and pants. Without such advice, patients could waste money on inappropriate aids or fail to understand how they work. Patients often have important questions about how to wear pads, how often to change them, and how to dispose of them: these can easily be answered by an experienced nurse.

Mild incontinence is often well contained by a simple pad (Fig. 10.1) or marsupial design pads and pants (Fig. 10.2). The advantage of the marsupial design is that the pad can be changed without the need to undress completely. Some degree of manual dexterity is needed, but carers can sometimes change the pads.

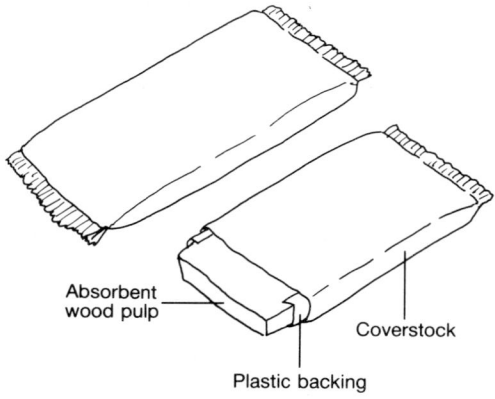

Absorbent wood pulp

Coverstock

Plastic backing

Fig. 10.1.   A simple incontinence pad.

If the patient has heavy incontinence or faecal soiling, then the system does not work. Some patients dislike handling the pads. An alternative for patients with light incontinence is a simple absorbent pad worn with normal underwear.

In severe urinary incontinence, pads and pants are the best answer (Fig. 10.3). Each pad has a water-repelling coverstock, absorbent material, and a plastic waterproof backing. Shaped pads containing virgin pulp, have performed well in tests.

All-in-one diapers (Fig. 10.4) are also used for severe incontinence but although they may effectively contain the

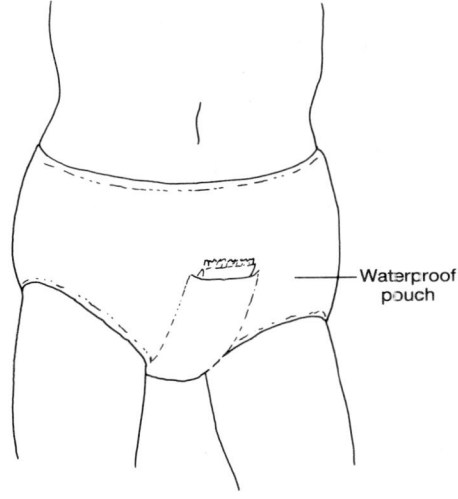

Fig. 10.2. Marsupial design pads and pants.

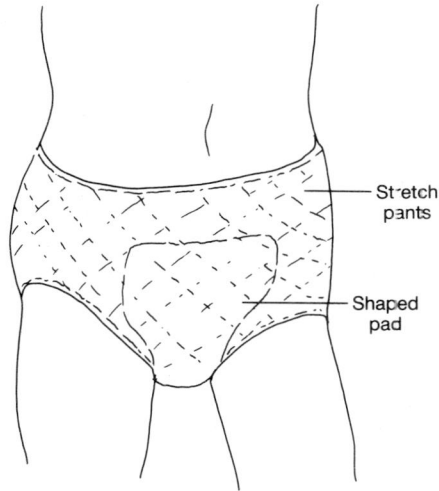

Fig. 10.3. Personally worn pads and pants.

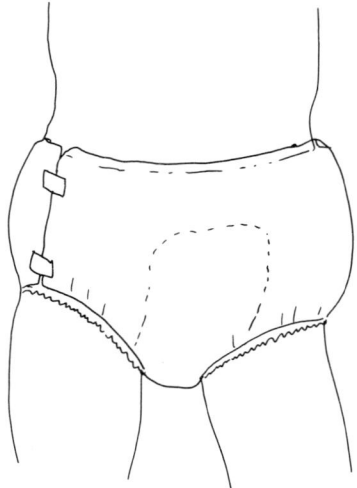

Fig. 10.4.   All-in-one adult diapers.

symptoms, some patients dislike the 'nappy design' and the patients are unable to change themselves unaided. They may occasionally be helpful for the patient with advanced dementia syndrome managed by a relative at home.

Frequent washing and changing of pads may help to prevent perineal rash, but some patients develop an urticarial rash in spite of scrupulous hygiene.

Nystatin will eradicate candidal infections; other approaches include changing to a different pad and pant system and using a milder washing powder for underwear.

People who use disposable pads will need to have a reliable method of disposing of the used pads. In some areas the Health Authority provides a 'black bag' collection system. Some patients, however, are sensitive to the stigma of putting extra bags outside the door for collection and having a special lorry to take them away and would rather make their own arrangements.

The most effective form of body-worn urine collection device for men is the penile sheath (Fig. 10.5). Penile sheaths which are self-adhesive or held in place by a latex strip are available on NHS prescription. Urine drains into a sterile leg bag in the same way as a catheter.

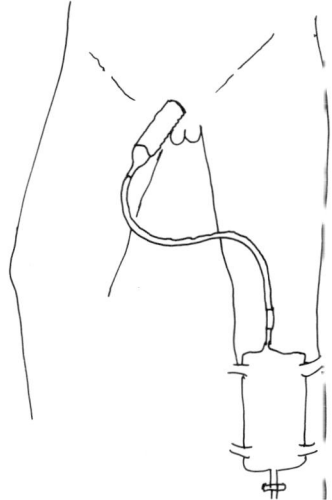

Fig. 10.5. Penile sheath and drainage system.

Once again, there is a need for careful explanation and fitting to ensure that the patient wears the correct size of sheath and reports any problems promptly.

Skin abrasions result from the sheath being pulled while urine stasis occurs if the drainage tube is kinked: both factors contribute to skin infections. It is important to discontinue using the sheath temporarily if such problems occur. In some males, penile retraction during the voiding reflex can be a problem. Although they are wearing the correct size of sheath, bypassing results from a reflex retraction of the penis when micturition is occurring.

Sometimes atrophy of the penis or a co-incidental inguinal hernia prevents any form of penile sheath from being effective.

An absorbent pouch can be helpful in containing post-micturition dribbling (Fig. 10.6). The penis fits into a lined pouch which is designed to absorb up to 100 ml. The pouch is held in place by an adhesive pad to the underpants.

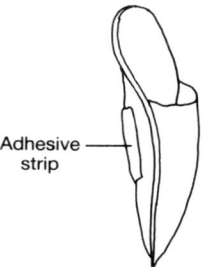

Adhesive
strip

Fig. 10.6.   An absorbent pouch for post-micturition dribbling.

The 'St. Peter's boat' is one example of a urinal designed for use by women confined to a wheelchair.

District nurses will be able to provide a list of contract and stock items available from the District Supplies Department. The District Supplies Office usually negotiate contract prices for the most commonly used pads and often provide nurse managers with details of the cost of each product.

A range of devices can be found at a growing number of disabled living centres all over the country. When visiting city-centre shops, a DIAL key allows the holder to use toilets adapted for disabled people.

11   Catheter management

Infection is the most important drawback to using a permanent catheter. All patients with a permanent catheter develop significant bacteriuria within a month of catheterization. Antibiotics only temporarily clear infection and prolonged courses are likely to breed resistant strains of bacteria.

Urinary tract infections can spread to cause: serious, life-threatening disease; progressive renal damage and pyelonephritis; acute epididymo-orchitis; and gram-negative septicaemia. Elderly patients are particularly at risk from septicaemia, which can be precipitated by minor procedures, such as changing a catheter.

It is not unusual for a confused elderly patient to pull a catheter out with the balloon inflated. The result is haematuria, followed a few days later by a severe pyrexial illness with rigors due to gram-negative septicaemia. Any patient who is liable to manipulate the catheter is better managed without.

A catheter specimen of urine (CSU) is not always a good guide to the infecting organism. The inside of a catheter provides a different environment for bacterial growth to the bladder wall and therefore supra-pubic aspirates commonly grow different organisms from the CSU.

Infections are a consequence of having a foreign body in the bladder and may be impossible to eradicate completely. Antiseptic washing of the perineum prior to catheterization does not eliminate the organisms in the distal urethra. These organisms may be advanced into the bladder when a catheter is inserted. The main route of invasion by bacteria is via the mucus around the catheter

which is secreted by urethral glands. Antibiotic impreg-
nation of catheters, cleaning of the urethral meatus, wash-
outs, antiseptic infusions, and acidifying the urine have no
effect on this route of infection.

Infection can be introduced each time the catheter is
separated from the urine bag, which breaks the closed
drainage system. Even when this is done to infuse anti-
septics, the result is an increase in infection rate. Patients
rarely tolerate infusions of noxyflex or chlorhexidine for
long enough to sterilize the urine.

For this reason, it is wise to avoid the use of spigots or
clamps designed to occlude the catheter when the bag is
disconnected. When bathing, for example, the catheter is
simply left connected to the leg bag which can be
unstrapped to wash the leg.

There is currently no laboratory test that will reliably
identify significant bacterial infection. There is some evidence that long-term catheters are associated with reflux of
urine into the renal pelvis, increasing the likelihood of
ascending infection.

Bladder pain, pyrexia, offensive urine or urethral dis-
charge are all indications for treatment in patients with a
positive CSU. The sensitivity report may help in suggesting
which antibiotic to prescribe. Trimethoprim and co-trimoxa-
zole are most frequently used as first-line treatments and
are relatively free from side-effects.

Multi-resistant organisms are often grown on culture.
Nitrofurantoin and nalidixic acid can be used, but they are
both expensive and likely to produce side-effects, such as
nausea, vomiting, rashes, and nitrofurantoin neuropathy.

Catheterization also results in loss of independence,
social stigma, pain or local discomfort, and catheter complications, such as blockage and bypassing. Female
patients who wear a dress or skirt find that the leg bag
invariably slips down to reveal their incontinence to
everyone. Many patients will be able to empty their own

leg bag and attach a night drainage bag in the evening but they may need assistance with catheter toilet or meatal cleaning.

Having a catheter often coincides with the end of an active sex life, but this need not be so; Sexual and Personal Relationships of the Disabled is an organization which publishes information for catheter users about sex (see Appendix).

Some catheterized patients complain of a constant pain or a continual sensation of needing to pass urine. The explanation probably lies in the sensitive area of the posterior urethra, which normally relaxes and fills with urine in the first step of the voiding reflex. Telling these patients to relax is often ineffective and many prefer to be managed without a catheter.

Other patients find that the catheter aggravates their unstable bladder, resulting in spasms of bladder pain due to powerful bladder contractions. Imipramine or terodiline can be given orally to control these attacks.

In spite of these drawbacks, a catheter can sometimes be highly effective in containing symptoms and keeping the patient dry.

Many catheterized patients develop blockage and bypassing. Oddly enough, larger catheters block and bypass more frequently than smaller ones. This is because a larger catheter is more likely to irritate the bladder wall and thus stimulate bladder contractions. Sometimes, large catheters are responsible for bladder spasms which are acutely uncomfortable to patients. The catheter is not like a plug in the bath; the urethra is immensely elastic but stretching it does not prevent catheter leakage and bypass.

The most important factors in blocking and bypassing are probably low fluid intake and urease-producing *Proteus* organisms. In theory, acidifying the urine should tip the balance away from *Proteus*, but attempts to achieve this using ascorbic acid have not been successful.

Twice-weekly infusions with, for example, Urimed Sub-agee may sometimes help to keep a catheter free from deposit: 100 ml of solution is run into the bladder through the main channel of the catheter. After 20 minutes, the solution is drained out again by placing the empty infusion bag below the level of the bladder.

Generally, 5 or 10 ml balloons probably cause less irritation of the bladder trigone but some patients with a lax urethra are unable to retain the smaller size and need a 30 ml balloon.

12   Developments in continence promotion

Continence promotion is an important aspect of health promotion which can be developed in general practice by a variety of methods:

- Further training of doctors and nurses
- Reviewing supplies of disposables
- Flagging and assessing patients
- Case-finding
- Clinical research

Further training

Although continence promotion features in some vocational training courses, there are no regular courses for doctors on this topic. The continence adviser may be able to help by giving lectures and working with the district nurses. There may be a local course on continence promotion which one of the district nurses could attend. The sector nurse manager will know if the ENB 978 course 'Promotion of continence and management of incontinence' is available locally. If a nurse in the practice is particularly interested, he/she may act as a link nurse, advising other nurses on first-line treatments and liaising with the continence adviser on their behalf.

Reviewing supplies

Some practices have introduced a record system to 'flag' patients receiving continence aids to ensure that they receive a periodic review. A simple card record system will provide information on trends in pads provided and average quantities per patient, which may be valuable in reviewing costs of providing disposables. A practice facilitator or manager may be able to take on some of the work of ordering and checking supplies of disposables.

Assessing patients

The continence adviser and the nurses can work together to introduce a system of assessment of all patients currently receiving pads and pants or using catheters. In some health districts, no pads are supplied without an assessment form completed by the patient's district nurse.

Christine Norton's book *Nursing for continence* summarizes the important points which should be included on an assessment form. Ideally, a thorough medical examination should be included.

Overall, the nurse's workload will increase as a result of promoting continence. Initially, less patients will need pads, but in time, more patients will present, so that eventually a larger number of patients will need supplies for incontinence. Although there are no savings in medical and nursing time, each patient that is improved or cured is extremely grateful and enjoys a much better quality of life as a result.

Case-finding

Only about half of the incontinent patients will be known to the practice. More patients may be encouraged to present by putting up a poster in the waiting room or sending out letters inviting patients with urinary symptoms to attend at particular times. Most patients with incontinence know that something is wrong and welcome the offer of investigation and treatment.

Simple, inexpensive treatments can be initiated in general practice and facilities for investigation and further treatment are developing rapidly as continence advisers are appointed in more health districts.

Some patients with incontinence only request treatment for other conditions, such as nervous disorders. Putting a poster in the waiting room may encourage them to present their real concern, incontinence, so that they can be fully assessed and treated.

Research

We understand so little about how incontinence presents and how effective treatment is that the field is wide open. Treatment of retention of urine is sure to be a major technique in medicine for the 1990s. New treatments for stress incontinence are being developed which need to be tried and tested, and we need to understand more about the psychology of incontinence and how best to use behavioural treatments. All of these topics are greatly in need of further study in general practice.

Appendix

Continence charts or information for patients about incontinence, pelvic floor exercises, intermittent self-catheterization, and indwelling catheters can be obtained from:

Bard Ltd, Pennywell Industrial Estate, Sunderland SR4 9EW

Coloplast Ltd, Peterborough Business Park, Peterborough PE2 0FX

EMS Medical Group Ltd, Unit 3, Stroud Industrial Estate,
    Stonedale Road, Oldends Lane, Stonehouse, Glos. GL10 2DG

Incare Medical Products, 43 Castle Street, Reading,
    Berks. RG1 7SN

Sexual and Personal Relationships of the Disabled, 286 Camden
    Road, London N7 0BJ

Simcare, Peter Road, Lancing, West Sussex BN15 8TJ

H. G. Wallace Ltd, Unit A, Commerce Way, Colchester,
    Essex CO2 8HH

The Bladderscan is a portable, battery-powered ultrasound device which measures bladder volume. It can be used by staff without any specialist radiological training after a short period of experience. Studies suggest that it is sensitive enough to identify significant urinary retention.

Further details are available from the UK distributors:
Lewis Medical, 826 Green Lanes, Winchmore Hill, London N21 2RT.

Bibliography

Association of Continence Advisors (1990). *Directory of continence aids.* Obtainable from: Association of Continence Advisors, 380-4 Harrow Road, London W9 2HU.

British Medical Association (1989). *Everyday aids and appliances.* Obtainable from: British Medical Journal, PO Box 295, London WC1H 9TE.

Department of Health and Social Services (1986). *Incontinence garments: Results of a DHSS study.* Health Equipment Information Vol. 159. Department of Health and Social Security, London.

Norton, C. (1986). *Nursing for continence.* Beaconsfield Publishers.

Roe, B. (1987). *Catheter care: A guide for users and their carers.* H. G. Wallace, Colchester.

Journal articles

Cardozo, L. D. and Stanton, S. L. (1980). Genuine stress incontinence and detrusor instability. *British Journal of Obstetrics and Gynaecology,* **87**, 184-90.

Castleden, C. M., George, C. F., Renwick, A. G., and Asher, M. J. (1981). Imipramine: a possible alternative to current therapy for urinary incontinence in the elderly. *Journal of Urology,* **125**, 318-20.

Castleden, C. M., Duffin, H. M., and Mitchell, E. P. (1984). Physiotherapy for stress incontinence. *Age and Ageing,* **13**, 235-7.

Castleden, C. M., Duffin, H. M., Asher, M. J., and Yeomanson, C. W. (1985). Factors influencing outcome in elderly patients with urinary incontinence and detrusor instability. *Age and Ageing,* **14**, 303-7.

Lancet Editorial (1986). Urinary incontinence in elderly patients. *Lancet,* **2**, 1316-17.

Lapides, J., Diokno, A. C., Silber, S. J., and Lowe, B. S. (1972). Clean intermittent self catheterisation in the management of urinary tract disease. *Journal of Urology*, **107**, 459-61.

McGrother, C. W., Castleden, C. M., Duffin, H., and Clarke, M. (1986). Provision of services for elderly incontinent people at home. *Journal of Epidemiology and Community Health*, **40**, 134-8.

Smith, N. K. G. (1988). Continence Advisory Services in England. *Health Trends*, **20**(1), 22-3.

Thomas, T. M., Plymat, K. R., Blannin, J., and Meade, T. W. (1980). Prevalence of urinary incontinence. *British Medical Journal*, **281**, 1243-5.

Whitelaw, G., Hammonds, J. C., and Tregellas, R. (1987). Clean intermittent self catheterisation in the elderly. *British Journal cf Urology*, **60**, 125-7.

Index